My Body Heals Itself.

Copyright Notice

Copyright © 2010 by James M. Wallace

All rights reserved. This book or any portion thereof may not be reproduced or used in any manner whatsoever without the express written permission of the publisher except for the use of brief quotations in a book review.

Table of contents

□□ **Becoming more aware of**

How Your Muscle are feeling and

How their connection to your Emotions can have

a positive Impact on your Overall Health. □□

Introduction

In our ever-changing world, it's easy to lose touch with our bodies. It's also easy to ignore the signals that our bodies are sending us. But our bodies are smart. They're smart enough to heal themselves. If we're paying attention, our bodies can heal themselves too.

Welcome to "My Body Heals Itself: becoming more aware of how your muscles are feeling and how they're connected to your emotions can impact your overall health."

In the next few pages, we'll take you on an exploration of how your emotions are connected to your muscles and how that connection affects your overall health. Have you ever noticed your neck and shoulders tighten when you're stressed? Or maybe you've experienced the calming effects of taking a deep breath and practicing mindfulness on the knots in your belly? These are just a few of how your emotions dance with your muscles. Your body's response to stress, happiness, sadness, and all other emotions is written in the tenseness and tenseness of your muscles.

The Importance of Understanding How Emotions Affect Our Physical Well-Being.

Emotions, an intricate tapestry of human emotion, have a powerful influence on our lives. Emotions have a major impact on shaping our bodily well-being, besides the apparent influence of mood and behavior. It's not an exaggeration to say that understanding the emotional impact on our physical health cannot be understated, since it reveals a holistic human existence in which brain and body are intimately connected.

Emotions are not limited to the realm of the mind; they reverberate throughout the body, creating a symphony of physiological responses. When we experience joy, our bodies can release endorphins, creating feelings of happiness and relaxation. Conversely, when faced with stress or fear, our bodies respond by activating the fight-or-flight response, releasing stress hormones such as cortisol and adrenaline. This response prepares us to respond quickly to perceived threats, but when chronic, it can be detrimental to our physical health.

Chronic stress, a common ailment in today's fast-paced world, highlights the profound connection between emotions and physical health. Prolonged exposure to stress hormones can lead to a range of health problems, including high blood pressure, weakened immune function, digestive problems, and cardiovascular disease. Understanding this connection requires us to take our mental health seriously because it directly affects our overall health and longevity.

In addition, emotions also have a significant influence on our immune system. Positive emotions like happiness and contentment have been shown to boost immune function, improving our ability to prevent disease. Conversely, negative emotions such as anger, anxiety, and sadness can weaken the immune system's defenses, making us more susceptible to infection and disease. Recognizing this connection highlights the importance of cultivating emotional resilience as the foundation of good health.

The impact of emotions on pain perception further highlights their role in physical health. Studies have found that people who maintain a positive attitude and practice relaxation techniques often experience reduced pain intensity. By altering our emotional state, we can effectively modulate our perception of pain, providing a powerful pain management tool.

In the field of chronic disease, the influence of emotions is especially important. Conditions like depression and anxiety often manifest with physical symptoms, including muscle tension, fatigue, and even cardiovascular problems. Treatment of these conditions often involves addressing the underlying emotional causes, emphasizing the inseparable connection between emotional and physical health.

Additionally, our emotional state can have a significant impact on our lifestyle choices, such as diet, exercise, and sleep. For example, emotional eating can lead to unhealthy eating habits, while chronic stress can prevent individuals from engaging in physical activity. These lifestyle choices in turn have direct consequences on our physical health. In short, understanding how emotions affect our physical health is essential to our overall health and quality of life. Emotions are not fleeting experiences limited to the mind; they are powerful forces that deeply affect our bodies. By recognizing this complex connection, we empower ourselves to take responsibility for our mental health as an integral part of our holistic health journey. Cultivating emotional resilience, managing stress, and maintaining positive emotions have become not only goals for their mental health but also essential strategies for maintaining and improving their physical health. ta. The importance of this connection reminds us that the path to optimal health includes both the mind and the body, and to truly thrive, we must care for both with equal dedication. together.

Chapter 1

The Mind-Body Connection

The Relationship Between Emotions and Muscles is Examined

Our journey begins by understanding the profound relationship between your emotions and your muscles. In this chapter, we will explore how your mind and body communicate, how past experiences shape your physical responses, and the science behind the mind-body connection.

The mind-body connection is not a new concept; it's been recognized for centuries in various cultures and healing practices. However, modern science has only recently begun to unravel the complex mechanisms at play. This chapter will provide you with a solid foundation for the chapters to come, offering a deeper understanding of the inner workings of your body.

The Concept of Mind-Body Connection

The mind-body link refers to the deep connection between a person's mental and emotional condition (the mind) and their physical health and well-being (the body). It implies that our ideas, emotions, and psychological experiences can substantially impact our physical health, and vice versa. This relationship is not simply a theoretical concept. It has long intrigued philosophers, scientists, and healers throughout history and has been widely explored and recognized in various professions, including medicine, psychology, and holistic health. Understanding and recognizing the mind-body link is critical for overall health and well-being. It emphasizes the importance of stress management, emotional well-being, and a holistic approach to healthcare that considers both mental and physical components.

The concept of mind-body connection is a fascinating exploration of the complex relationship between our thoughts, emotions, and physical health. It delves deeper into the idea that our mental and emotional state can have a profound impact on our physiological health and vice versa.

At its core, the mind-body connection is based on the understanding that our thoughts, emotions, and mental state have a direct impact on our physical health and vice versa. This concept recognizes that the human body is a complex and interconnected system in which the mental and emotional aspects are intimately linked to the physical. This shows that the thoughts we think and the emotions we feel can trigger physiological responses in our bodies.

One of the fundamental pillars of the mind-body connection is the recognition that stress, anxiety, and other negative emotions can manifest physically. For example, when we experience stress, our bodies respond by releasing stress hormones such as cortisol and adrenaline. This physiological response prepares us for the "fight or flight" response, which can be life-saving in an emergency but detrimental when prolonged. Chronic stress is linked to a range of health problems, from heart disease to digestive disorders, highlighting the complex connection between our emotional state and physical health.

Conversely, positive emotions such as happiness, gratitude, and love can provide profound health benefits. Studies have shown that people with a positive outlook on life tend to have stronger immune systems, lower blood pressure, and a reduced risk of chronic diseases. The mind-body connection emphasizes that cultivating a positive mindset can contribute to overall well-being.

Additionally, the mind-body connection extends to the realm of cognition and pain management. Practicing mindfulness, meditation, and relaxation techniques have been used as powerful tools for pain relief. By shifting attention from pain to a state of calm and relaxation, individuals can effectively reduce the intensity of pain sensations. This demonstrates the mind's ability to regulate physical sensations.

The concept of connecting mind and body is not limited to the treatment of physical ailments. It also has profound implications for mental health. For example, people with depression and anxiety often experience physical symptoms such as muscle tension and fatigue. By addressing the root causes of emotions, therapy, and counseling can alleviate mental and physical suffering, demonstrating the bidirectional nature of this connection.

Chapter 2

Muscle Memory

How Past Events Influence How Your Body Reacts

In the previous chapter, we explored the intricate relationship between your emotions and your muscles. Now, let's take a closer look at how your past experiences shape your body's responses, creating what we commonly refer to as "muscle memory."

Your ability to recall how to ride a bike or play an instrument is just the tip of the iceberg of the amazing phenomenon known as muscle memory. The way your body responds to stress and emotions is another important aspect of it. In addition to physical prowess, your muscles may also recall emotional memories.

Think of a time in the past when you had tremendous fear or worry. It can have been a close call while driving, a speaking engagement in front of an audience, or a traumatic experience. Your body stiffened up in those circumstances as a result of the fight-or-flight response, an instinctive response created to defend you.

Now, think about how your body responds when you recall those memories or encounter similar situations. Although there is no imminent physical threat, you could observe that your muscles still contract similarly. This is an example of your body's muscle memory.

To better understand our bodies and emotions, we must first understand muscle memory. We can start to understand the relationship between our minds and muscles by observing how previous experiences influence our physical responses. Gaining more control over our body and, ultimately, our mental well-being starts with awareness.

In the next chapters, we'll look at methods and exercises that can help you let go of and rewire your muscle memory so you can react to stress and emotions in healthier ways. We'll also examine the importance of relaxation and how it helps to end the cycle of muscular tension. So, pay attention as we continue to unlock the mysteries of your body's remarkable capacity for self-healing.

Chapter 3

The Power of Relaxation

How to Reduce Muscle Tension

In the previous chapters, we explored the intricate relationship between your emotions and muscles, as well as the concept of muscle memory. It's time to explore the transforming potential of relaxation practices. You may relax your muscles, end the cycle of stress, and improve your overall well-being by using these techniques.

In our fast-paced lives, stress has become a common companion. It can cause persistent muscle tension, which in turn may make mental misery worse. The good news is that by relaxing, you can break this cycle.

Relaxation isn't just about lying on a beach or taking a spa day (although those can be quite rejuvenating). It's a deliberate practice that can be incorporated into your daily routine, helping you manage stress and cultivate a sense of inner calm. When you relax your muscles, you send a signal to your brain that it's safe to let go of tension, and this, in turn, can influence your emotional state.

This chapter will cover a variety of relaxation methods, such as progressive muscle relaxation, mindfulness meditation, and deep breathing exercises. These techniques are made to make you more conscious of your muscular stress and give you the means to relieve it.

Deep breathing is one of the easiest yet most powerful practices. You can cause your body to relax by inhaling slowly and deeply. Deep breathing helps your muscles receive more oxygen, which eases tension and encourages relaxation. We'll walk you through particular breathing techniques you can use every day.

A further effective technique is progressive muscular relaxation. This method entails sequentially tensing and then relaxing various bodily muscle groups. By practicing this, you increase your awareness of muscle tension and learn how to purposefully release it. It's a routine that might relieve stress or prepare you for sleep.

This chapter will also include mindfulness meditation. Being entirely in the present, without passing judgment, is the essence of mindfulness. You can become attentive to your body's sensations, such as muscle tightness, and learn to let it go. Breaking the cycle of stress and emotional reactivity can be facilitated by this technique.

You'll learn practical methods that you can use right now as we delve further into each relaxation technique. These methods will not only assist you in relaxing your muscles but will also enhance your general emotional well-being. Keep in mind that your body has a great capacity for self-healing and that one of the keys to releasing this potential is relaxation.

In brief, here are some practical strategies for mindful meditation:

- **Find a Quiet Place**: For meditation, choose a tranquil, clutter-free location.

- **Comfortable Posture**: Sit or lie down in a position that is comfortable for you.

- **Pay Attention to Your Breathing**: Pay attention to your breathing. Exhale and inhale normally.

- **Observe Ideas:** Acknowledge thoughts without judgment, then return to your breath softly.

- **Body Scan**: Mentally scan your body, recognizing and releasing any tension.

- **Sensory Awareness**: Pay attention in the current moment to sounds, sensations, and odors.

- **Set a timer**: Begin with a short duration and progressively increase as you gain confidence.

- **Practice on a regular basis**: Consistency is essential. To reap the full benefits of mindfulness, aim for daily meditation.

To find the way to a healthier, more balanced life, let's start this adventure of relaxation and self-healing.

Chapter 4

Stress and Its Impact on Muscles

Breaking the Cycle of Stress and Muscle Damage

In the preceding chapters, we've explored the intricate connection between your emotions and muscles, the concept of muscle memory, and the transformative power of relaxation techniques. Let's now discuss how to stop the cycle of tension as well as the deep effects stress has on your muscles.

Although it occasionally acts as a motivator or a protector, stress is an inevitable aspect of life and can have negative effects on your physical and mental well-being. Muscle tightness is one of the most typical physical signs of stress.

Your body's natural reaction to stress, whether it's brought on by work, relationships, or other demands in your life, is to tense up in anticipation of a threat. The body's "fight or flight" reaction, which is intended to help you respond swiftly in potentially dangerous situations, includes this muscular tension. However, persistent stress can cause your muscles to stay tense for an extended time, resulting in discomfort, pain, and even emotional suffering.

We'll examine the mechanics underlying stress-related muscular tension in this chapter to better understand how your body responds to stress. We'll also discuss the negative effects of ongoing stress on your physical and mental health.

But comprehending stress is just the beginning. Understanding how to control and reduce muscle tension brought on by stress is where the true power lies. We'll cover a wide range of useful approaches that you may apply in your everyday life, from stress-reduction methods like mindfulness and exercise to lifestyle adjustments that encourage calm.

We'll also go over how crucial it is to create boundaries, use time wisely, and get social support to lessen stress in your life. You may stop the cycle of tension and open the door to increased physical and emotional well-being by attacking stress from many sides.

Remember that when given the correct resources and assistance, your body has an amazing capacity to cure itself. You can make substantial progress toward releasing your body's innate healing capacity by comprehending stress and how it affects your muscles and putting those insights into practice.

Follow along as we investigate the relationship between stress and muscle tension and let's work together to end the cycle of ongoing stress.

Chapter 5

The Healing Touch

Massage and Its Therapeutic Benefits

We have looked into muscle memory, relaxation methods, and the consequences of stress in our quest to understand the connection between emotions and muscles and how it affects your general health. Let's now explore the art of massage, which is a highly therapeutic element of healing.

Since ancient times, massage has been a potent technique for fostering both physical and mental well-being. It's more than simply a fancy spa treatment; it's a routine that has a significant impact on your emotional stability and muscle health.

In this chapter, we'll explore the therapeutic advantages of massage and how it can help you relax, relieve stress, and feel better overall. Whether or whether you've had a professional massage, this chapter will provide you with insightful knowledge about the power of touch to heal.

Massage therapy involves exerting pressure on the body's soft tissues, including the muscles and connective tissues, and manipulating them. This physical manipulation has several advantageous outcomes:

1. **Muscle Relaxation**: Skilled massage therapists can locate tight muscles and use specific techniques to remove that tension, increasing relaxation and providing relief from sore muscles.

2. **Reduction of Stress**: The slow, rhythmic movements of massage can start the body's relaxation response, which lowers the levels of stress chemicals in your body.

3. **Improved Circulation**: Massage increases blood flow, which helps your muscles receive more oxygen and nutrients and can help with healing and inflammation reduction.

4. **Enhanced Mood**: Endorphins released during a massage can improve your mood and foster a sense of well-being.

5. **Emotional Release**: For many people, massage therapy provides a secure setting in which to let go of repressed feelings and trauma that the body may be holding onto.

This chapter will discuss several massage techniques, from Swedish to deep tissue and beyond, each of which has its special advantages. You'll discover how to select the best kind of massage for your unique requirements and preferences.

Even though professional massages are quite helpful, we'll also go over massage techniques that you may use at home or while on the road to relieve stress and muscular tightness.

Here's a brief overview of some common massage techniques and their distinct benefits:

1. Swedish massage

   - Strokes that are gentle and calming.

   - Reduces tension and improves circulation.

   - Ideal for total relaxation.

2. Deep Tissue Massage

   - Firm pressure is used to target deeper muscle levels.

   - Chronic pain and muscle strain are relieved.

   - Beneficial for athletes and people dealing with special challenges.

3. Hot Stone Massage

   - Muscles are relaxed by using warm stones.

   - Deep relaxation and stress alleviation are promoted.

- Ideal for improving general well-being.

4. Aromatherapy Massage

- Massage is combined with essential oils.

- It promotes relaxation and can be used to address specific issues.

- Provides a sensory experience to aid with emotional balance.

5. Sports Massage

- Athletes and energetic people benefit from sports massage.

- Dedicated to the prevention and treatment of sports-related injuries.

- Improves performance and adaptability.

6. Thai Massage

- Stretching and yoga-like movements are used in Thai massage.

- Flexibility, balance, and energy flow are all improved.

- Encourages overall physical well-being.

A massage is an opportunity for self-care and self-awareness, so keep in mind that it's more than just a physical sensation. You can take advantage of your body's intrinsic capacity for healing and achieve harmony between your physical and emotional well-being by including massage in your health regimen.

So, whether you're a novice or an experienced enthusiast, join us as we explore the tremendous therapeutic advantages of this ancient healing practice in Chapter 5.

Chapter 6

Yoga and Stretching

Regaining Connection to Your Body

We now focus on stretching and yoga techniques as we continue to investigate the complex interaction between emotions and muscles. These techniques provide an effective way to re-establish a connection with your body, encourage flexibility, and improve both your physical and emotional well-being.

Yoga is a holistic practice that incorporates breathing exercises, mindful breathing, meditation, and physical postures. It has been practiced for a very long time and is famous for its capacity to foster physical toughness, flexibility, and mental clarity. Increasing one's awareness of one's body and emotions is another important benefit of yoga.

We will explore the advantages of yoga and stretching in this chapter, learning how they help reduce stress and tension while enhancing mobility and instilling a sense of inner tranquility.

Yoga: A Way to Find Balance in Your Body and Mind

Yoga is a holistic method of treatment that takes into account both the body and the mind. Yoga works to relax tight muscles, enhance posture, and raise general body awareness through a series of poses and movements.

The emphasis on the mind-body connection is one of the distinctive features of yoga. You are urged to focus on your breath and physical feelings as you proceed through the yoga poses. By practicing mindfulness, you can learn to be more aware of how your body reacts to various feelings and circumstances.

Stretching: Improving Flexibility and Reducing Tension

Another effective technique for strengthening your connection to your body and enhancing muscular health is stretching. Regular stretching exercises can enhance your range of motion, decrease muscular tension, and promote flexibility. Your muscles are less likely to become stiff and uncomfortable when you are more flexible.

We'll walk you through a variety of stretching and yoga poses in this chapter that you may include in your everyday practice. These techniques can assist you in releasing muscle tension, enhancing your physical well-being, and increasing your awareness of the mind-body connection, regardless of your level of experience.

Without a doubt, here is a short collection of stretching and yoga poses for your everyday practice:

- **Child's Pose**: A resting posture to stretch and relax the back.
- **Downward Dog**: It is a full-body stretch that strengthens the arms and legs.

- **Cobra Pose**: Stretches the spine and opens the chest.

- **Warrior Pose**: This pose strengthens the legs and promotes balance.

- **Tree Pose:** Improves balance and concentration.

- **Cat-Cow Stretch:** Mobilizes and stretches the spine.

- **Seated Forward Bend:** Stretches the hamstrings and back while seated.

- **Bridge Pose:** This posture strengthens the back and glutes.

- **Pigeon Pose:** This stretch opens the hips and relieves tension.

- **Corpse Pose:** A last rest and rejuvenation pose.

Incorporate these poses into your everyday routine to increase flexibility, decrease tension, and enhance general well-being.

Join us on this yoga and stretching adventure to find your body. You'll improve your physical flexibility and develop a deeper knowledge of how your emotions are closely related to your physical experiences by adopting these routines into your life.

We'll keep talking about how to use the mind-body connection to enhance your health and well-being in the chapters that follow.

Chapter 7

Nutrition for Muscle Health

What You Need to Know

We now turn our attention to nutrition, a crucial component of health that has a significant impact on both your emotional balance and the health of your muscles, in our quest to comprehend the intricate relationship between emotions, muscles, and overall health.

You are what you eat, according to the adage. Your diet is crucial in giving your muscles the nutrition they require to operate at their peak. Additionally, it may affect your emotional health, energy level, and mood.

This chapter will examine the crucial part that nutrition plays in maintaining both emotional stability and muscle health. We'll go into detail on the nutrients your muscles need, the relationship between a healthy diet and your emotions, and useful dietary tips to promote both your physical and mental well-being.

The Foundation of Muscle Health

For your muscles to work properly, they need a number of different nutrients. For instance, protein is necessary for muscle growth and repair. The maintenance of muscle tissue depends heavily on amino acids, which are the building blocks of protein. We'll go over ways to acquire enough protein in your diet and look into plant-based protein options for people who live vegetarian or vegan lifestyles.

Another essential element for the health of muscles is carbohydrates. They supply the energy your muscles require to work effectively. We'll discuss the distinctions between complex and simple carbohydrates and how to choose nutritious carbs that will support your energy levels and muscular performance.

In addition, vitamins and minerals including vitamin D, calcium, magnesium, and potassium are crucial for maintaining healthy muscles. We'll talk about ways to make sure you're getting enough of these micronutrients to support healthy muscle function as well as their roles and dietary sources.

Emotional eating and nutritious eating

Beyond the physical, eating has a significant impact on your emotional health as well. Emotional eating, or using food to deal with emotions, is a widespread behavior. A vital first step in developing a positive relationship with food is realizing how your emotions and eating behaviors are related.

We'll discuss the idea of mindful eating, which entails being aware of your hunger cues, appreciating your meals, and making deliberate decisions regarding what you eat. By engaging in mindful eating, you can improve your ability to control emotional eating and cultivate a healthy relationship with food.

Practical Nutritional Techniques

We'll offer useful nutritional advice that you may use in your daily life to wrap up this chapter. With the use of these techniques, you may support the health of your muscles, maintain emotional equilibrium, and lay the groundwork for long-term wellness and vitality.

The information and methods in this chapter will help you make wise food decisions that are good for your body and your emotions, whether you're trying to improve your mood, maximize your muscular performance, or just eat more thoughtfully.

So come along as we investigate how nutrition has a significant impact on both emotional stability and muscle health. You can advance significantly on your path to better general health by feeding your body with intention and awareness.

Making good dietary choices in your everyday life is important not just for your physical health but also for your mental well-being. Choosing the appropriate nutrition can help you feel better, perform better in the gym, and eat more mindfully.

- Begin by emphasizing complete, unprocessed foods. Fruits, vegetables, lean proteins, and whole grains are high in vitamins, minerals, and antioxidants, which help your body as well as your emotions. These foods give continuous energy, lower inflammation, and improve overall health.

- Pay attention to portion amounts as well. Mindful eating can help you maintain a healthy weight and avoid overeating, which can cause emotional pain and muscle strain.

- Drink plenty of water throughout the day. Dehydration can have an impact on your emotions and physical performance. Drinking enough water promotes muscle function and cognitive clarity.

- Consider eating foods high in tryptophan, such as turkey and tofu, as well as those high in omega-3 fatty acids, such as salmon and flaxseeds. These can have a favorable impact on your emotional state.

- Finally, don't overlook the significance of balance. Treat yourself on occasion, but make sure your overall diet is well-balanced and full of healthful options.

Chapter 8

Exercise and Endorphins

Elevating Your Mood Naturally

Our exploration into the complex relationship between feelings, muscles, and general health now turns to exercise and its unique capacity to elevate your mood in a completely natural way by releasing endorphins.

Exercise is a powerful tool for enhancing emotional well-being and preserving a healthy mind-body balance. It is not simply about improving physical fitness. The science underlying how exercise impacts your mood, the kinds of physical activities that can improve your spirits, and how to incorporate regular exercise into your life for maximum benefits are all covered in this chapter.

The Endorphin Relationship

Exercise has a profoundly positive impact on one's emotional state thanks in large part to endorphins, also known as "feel-good" hormones. Your body releases endorphins during physical activity, which are organic painkillers and mood enhancers. Your brain's receptors are affected by these neurotransmitters to lessen pain perception and foster feelings of happiness and well-being.

Knowing how exercise affects endorphins is essential because it brings to light the significant emotional impact that exercise may have. Regular exercise can boost happiness, lessen the effects of depression and anxiety, and act as a natural stress-relieving mechanism.

Picking the Best Exercise

When it comes to boosting mood, not all forms of exercise are made equal. We will look at many forms of exercise and how they can affect our mental health in particular:

Exercise that increases your heart rate and breathing is referred to as aerobic exercise. They are well known for boosting mood and can be especially helpful in lowering stress and anxiety.

Strength Training: Adding muscle increases mental well-being by boosting self-esteem and body confidence in addition to physical strength.

Yoga and mind-body exercises integrate physical postures with mindfulness and breath awareness to promote both physical and emotional well-being.

Outdoor Activities: Engaging in outdoor activities like riding or hiking where you can connect with nature can be incredibly calming and uplifting.

Making Exercise a Part of Your Routine

It takes ambition and dedication to make fitness a regular part of your life. Even if you have a busy schedule, we'll provide you with useful advice on how to include exercise in your daily routine.

Here's a technique for making exercise a non-negotiable part of your hectic schedule.

- Plan and prioritize your tasks.

The first step is to acknowledge the value of exercise in your overall health. Physical activity on a regular basis benefits your physical health, mental clarity, and stress management. It's a worthwhile investment in yourself.

Begin by establishing specific, attainable goals. Understand your goals for exercising, whether they be to improve fitness, reduce stress, or increase energy levels.

- Make an appointment for it.

Exercise should be treated as you would any other appointment or commitment in your day. Make clear time slots for your workouts that are non-negotiable. This method helps you see exercise as a necessary element of your routine rather than an optional extra. Discover and choose activities you enjoy, create reasonable fitness goals, and get through typical roadblocks that might be keeping you from being active.

- Short and Intense Workouts

To keep fit, you don't need to spend hours at the gym. Short, targeted exercises and high-intensity interval training (HIIT) can deliver considerable advantages in a shorter time frame. These workouts are quick and easy to execute, taking around 20-30 minutes.

- Include It in Your Daily Activities

Look for ways to incorporate fitness into your regular routine. Choose stairs over elevators, walk or cycle to work if possible, and take a quick stroll during your lunch hour. These minor adjustments might build up over time.

- Multitasking

Make the most of your time by adding exercise into things you currently perform. You can, for example, conduct bodyweight exercises while watching TV, take phone conversations while walking, or hold a walking meeting at work.

- Intensity trumps consistency.

Making exercise a habit requires consistency. It is preferable to undertake a shorter, lower-intensity workout on a regular basis rather than sporadic severe bouts. Set realistic goals and progressively raise the intensity over time.

- Mentality and Accountability

It is critical to keep a positive attitude and hold yourself accountable. To keep motivated, consider finding an exercise partner or enrolling in a fitness class. Tracking your progress and appreciating minor triumphs might help you stay motivated.

- Adapt to Your Schedule

Recognize that your routine may alter, and that is just fine. Be versatile and open to change your workout routine as needed. Consistency is essential, but flexibility in how and when you exercise is also essential.

You'll have a thorough understanding of how exercise can innately improve your mood and foster emotional well-being by the end of this chapter.

Exercise isn't simply good for your body; it's also a great mood enhancer. Here's how it's done:

1. Endorphins, dopamine, and serotonin are released during exercise, which lifts your mood.

2. Stress Reduction: It lowers cortisol (the stress hormone), making you more tolerant to stress.

3. Improved Sleep: Regular exercise increases sleep quality, which is essential for emotional well-being.

4. Self-esteem and self-confidence are enhanced when fitness goals are met.

5. Emotional Release: Exercise aids in the release of pent-up emotions and promotes emotional balance.

6. Group activities strengthen social bonds and provide emotional support.

7. Mindfulness: Yoga and other mindfulness practices promote self-awareness and emotional regulation.

Design an exercise program that complements your tastes and fits into your lifestyle.

So come along as we explore the amazing effects of exercise on your mood and general health. It's time to use movement to improve your mood and build a more satisfying and balanced existence.

Chapter 9

Breathwork

Unlocking Emotional Release through Breathing

We now focus on breathwork, a transformative practice that enables you to access the power of your breath to unlock emotional release, lessen muscle tension, and promote inner peace. As we continue on our quest to understand the profound relationship between emotions, muscles, and well-being, breathwork will become an increasingly important part of our discussion.

In our daily lives, breathing is a vital but frequently ignored process. Breathwork can have a significant positive impact on your emotional and physical health, even though we frequently take it for granted.

The skill of conscious breathing, its effects on your muscles and emotions, and numerous breathwork techniques that can assist in releasing tension and restoring emotional balance are all covered in this chapter.

Breath, Mind, and Body Connection

Your breath serves as a link between your body and mind. Your breathing pattern alters when you're upset or concerned, frequently becoming shallow and fast. Your body then receives the signal to maintain its state of high alert, which causes tension in your muscles and emotional distress.

On the other hand, when you practice conscious, deep breathing, you tell your brain that it's okay to unwind. This causes the release of chemicals that promote relaxation, which can help lower stress levels, alleviate tension in the muscles, and promote calmness.

Breathing Exercises

We'll go over several methods for breathwork that you can use every day, including:

- **Deep Breathing**: Simple yet incredibly efficient, deep breathing involves taking slow, deliberate breaths to calm your nervous system and reduce stress.

- **Diaphragmatic Breathing**: This technique focuses on using your diaphragm to breathe deeply, promoting better oxygenation and relaxation.

- **Box breathing**: A method for resetting your neurological system that involves breathing in, holding, exhaling, and holding in equal numbers.

- **Pranayama**: A variety of breath control exercises that are descended from yoga and can help you control your emotions and energy are known as pranayama techniques.

Unlocking Emotional Release

Allowing for emotional release through breathwork is one of its most potent features. Tension in your muscles can be a sign of unreleased emotions. You can connect with these feelings and then let them out in a safe, regulated way utilizing breathwork, which aids in emotional healing and general well-being.

Breath Awareness Meditation: A mindfulness practice that involves observing your breath without trying to change it. Your self-awareness and emotional control may improve as a result.

Follow along as we explore breathwork and together let's unleash the breath's transforming power.

Chapter 10

Visualization and Mindfulness

Harnessing the Mind-Body Connection

We are now moving into the areas of visualization and mindfulness in our investigation of the complex relationship between emotions, muscles, and general health. This is an investigation of the ability of your mind to affect your physical and emotional well-being.

A significant and much-underused component of self-healing is the mind-body link. You can use visualization and mindfulness to tap into this link, which helps with muscle relaxation, emotional stability, and overall wellness.

The ideas of visualization and mindfulness, their effects on your muscles and emotions, and useful methods you can employ to incorporate these practices into your daily life are all covered in this chapter.

The Influence of Vision

Using your mind to conjure up scenarios or mental images is a technique called visualization. It can significantly improve both your physical and emotional well-being when used mindfully. This is how:

- **Muscle Relaxation**: You can tell your muscles to release tension by picturing yourself in a relaxed condition. This is particularly useful for releasing stiff muscles brought on by tension.

- **Stress reduction**: Using visualization techniques will help you enter a peaceful and tranquil state of mind, which can lessen your stress level and improve your emotional well-being.

- **Positive affirmations**: Repeating happy phrases and visualizing positive results can improve your emotional well-being and boost your self-assurance and self-esteem.

Mindfulness: Being Present in the Moment

Being completely present in the now, without passing judgment, is the discipline of mindfulness. Being mindful allows you to be more aware of your body's feelings, thoughts, and sensations. Your emotional and physical health may be significantly affected by this awareness:

- **Muscle Tension Awareness**: Using mindfulness, you can become more conscious of your muscles as they tense up, allowing you to relax them deliberately.

- **Emotional Regulation**: By learning to observe your emotions objectively and respond to them in better ways, you can lessen emotional distress.

- **Reducing Stress**: Mindfulness techniques, like meditation and focused breathing, trigger the relaxation response, which lowers stress hormones and fosters serenity.

Practical Visualization and Mindfulness Techniques

We will investigate useful methods for both mindfulness and visualization, such as:

- **Guided Imagery**: A technique for visualization in which you follow a written or audio script as it leads you on a calming mental journey.

- **Meditation**: Mindfulness meditation techniques that support the development of awareness and present-moment attention.

- **Body Scans**: You can locate and relieve tension in your muscles by deliberately focusing your attention on various sections of your body.

Let's explore visualization and mindfulness together as we move closer to deeper self-awareness and inner serenity.

Chapter 11

Emotional Release Techniques

Letting Go for Healing

We now dig into the area of emotional release techniques as part of our ongoing investigation into the complex relationship between emotions, muscles, and general well-being. This is an exploration of how to let go of suppressed emotions, lessen muscle tension, and promote healing.

Your physical health is strongly influenced by your emotions, and unresolved emotional difficulties can show up as stiffness and discomfort in your muscles. You may improve your emotional and physical well-being by learning how to process and properly release your emotions.

This chapter will cover a variety of emotional release techniques, their effects on muscle health, and useful techniques for letting go and healing.

Emotional Stress and Muscle Tension

Being intimately related to your body, emotions are not independent experiences. As part of the fight-or-flight response, your body frequently tenses up your muscles in response to strong emotions like anger, grief, or anxiety. If emotions are not properly handled, this tension can persist for extended periods, resulting in discomfort and agony.

The first step in realizing the value of emotional release is to comprehend the relationship between emotions and physical tension. You can stop the cycle of muscle tension and find comfort both physically and emotionally by addressing unresolved emotions.

Techniques for Releasing Emotions

We'll look at a few methods for letting emotions go:

- **Writing in a journal**: can be a therapeutic way to process and let go of bottled-up emotions.

- **Artistic Expression**: Engaging in creative activities like painting, drawing, or sculpting can provide a non-verbal outlet for emotions.

- **Therapeutic strategies**: You can explore and let go of buried emotions using methods like talk therapy and somatic therapy.

- **Breathwork**: As was mentioned in earlier chapters, breathwork is a potent method for letting go of emotions that have been held in the body.

- **The techniques of mindfulness and meditation**: can provide a secure environment where emotions can be acknowledged and let go of without fear of repercussion.

Practical Techniques for Release of Emotions

You can process and let go of emotions as they come with the help of the useful strategies, we'll give you to adopt into your daily life. Additionally, you'll discover how to spot emotional red flags and create effective coping skills for dealing with strong emotions.

Chapter 12

Pain Management

Strategies to Alleviate Muscle Discomfort

We now concentrate on pain management—an exploration of methods to relieve muscular discomfort and enhance your physical and mental health—as we continue our investigation into the delicate relationship between emotions, muscles, and general well-being.

Muscle strain, stress, and unresolved emotions are just a few of the things that can cause discomfort and pain in the muscles. Understanding the causes of muscle pain and giving you useful pain management techniques are the main goals of this chapter.

Understanding the Causes of Muscle Pain

Understanding the causes of muscular discomfort is crucial before discussing pain management techniques:

- Tension in muscles Chronic pain can result from persistent muscle tension, which is frequently brought on by stress or emotional issues.

- Physical overuse: Exercising excessively or performing physical labor can make your muscles sore and uncomfortable.

- Injury: Muscle discomfort and stiffness can result from acute injuries or repetitive strain injuries.

- Unresolved feelings and tension can emerge physically as aches and pains in the muscles.

Pain Control Techniques

We'll examine many pain-reduction techniques to ease muscle discomfort:

- Exercises to Increase Flexibility and Stretching: Stretching exercises that are done gently can relieve muscle tension.

- Physical therapy: Using specific exercises and procedures, a physical therapist can help with muscle pain and stiffness.

- Regular massages and bodywork sessions can help ease discomfort and reduce muscle tension.

- Hot and Cold Therapy: Muscle discomfort and inflammation can be reduced by applying heat or cold to the affected area.

- Non-prescription painkillers can be used to treat mild to moderate muscle pain. These medications are available over-the-counter.

- Mind-Body Methods: Methods like meditation, mindfulness, and guided visualization can ease discomfort and muscle tension.

- Nutrition: Eating a well-balanced diet that includes items that fight inflammation will improve muscular health and lessen discomfort.

- Muscle pain can be subtly reduced by practicing stress management strategies like deep breathing, meditation, and yoga.

Creating a Personalized Pain Management Plan

Muscle discomfort is a distinct sensation for each person. We will assist you in creating a specialized pain treatment strategy that takes into account your unique requirements, preferences, and the underlying reasons for your muscular discomfort.

By the end of this chapter, you'll have a thorough understanding of the causes of muscular pain and a toolset of pain-relieving techniques to help you feel better overall. Join us on this pain management journey, and let's collaborate to design a life that is less painful and more comfortable.

Understanding Muscular Pain Causes and Creating a Pain-Relief Toolkit

Muscular discomfort is a common, often severe condition that many of us may encounter at some point in our lives. It can be caused by a variety of conditions, such as physical strain, injury, stress, or even emotional problems. It is critical to acquire a toolkit of pain-relieving techniques and a full awareness of the causes of muscular pain in order to properly manage and alleviate it. This all-encompassing strategy not only alleviates immediate discomfort but also contributes to a greater overall sense of well-being.

Understanding Muscular Pain Causes:

- Overexertion: Overexertion is a typical cause of muscular pain. Strenuous exercise, hard lifting, or bad posture can all cause this. Understanding your body's limits and practicing correct ergonomics might help prevent such suffering.

- Muscle pain can be caused by accidents, falls, or sports-related injuries. It is critical to recognize the indicators of injury and get appropriate medical attention.

- Emotional Stress: Physical symptoms of emotional stress include muscle stiffness and soreness. When you are stressed or concerned, your body responds by tightening muscles. Chronic tension can result in chronic discomfort.

Creating a Pain-Relief Toolbox:

- Pain Management Techniques: It is critical to learn how to handle pain. This covers methods such as using heat or cold therapy to relieve acute pain or practicing relaxation exercises to relieve persistent tension.

- Regular stretching and exercise regimens can improve flexibility and muscular strength, lowering the chance of pain.

- Massage therapy can target specific areas of pain and provide relief by relaxing stiff muscles.

- Mind-Body Techniques: Through relaxation and self-awareness, techniques such as mindfulness, yoga, and meditation can help you become more attuned to your body and manage pain.

- Nutrition: A well-balanced diet rich in anti-inflammatory foods can help improve overall muscle health. Pain relievers, whether over-the-counter or prescribed, can be used when necessary, but should be taken with caution and under expert supervision.

- Professional Assistance: Seeking medical guidance or talking with a physical therapist can provide specialized remedies for your individual situation if your pain is severe or persistent.

You can better manage and eliminate discomfort by establishing a toolkit of pain-relieving strategies and knowing the origins of musculoskeletal pain. Furthermore, this all-encompassing method not only relieves the present discomfort but also improves your entire well-being. It gives you the ability to take care of your health and live a life with less discomfort and higher quality of life.

Chapter 13

Holistic Healing

Integrating Body, Mind, and Emotions

We are now embarking on a journey of holistic healing—an exploration of how to integrate your body, mind, and emotions for a more balanced and peaceful life—as part of our continuous investigation into the complex relationship between emotions, muscles, and general well-being.

Your physical, emotional, and mental states are interrelated, and a holistic healing approach acknowledges this. You may encourage maximum well-being and a greater comprehension of the mind-body relationship by encouraging harmony among these factors.

The Holistic Method of Healthcare

Holistic health recognizes that your body and mind are connected components of a whole rather than two distinct entities. The other aspects of your existence may be impacted if one of them is out of harmony. Unresolved emotions, for instance, might cause physical tension and discomfort, and the latter can affect how you're feeling emotionally.

We'll look at the fundamentals of holistic healing in this chapter and see how they might be used to lead a well-rounded, integrated existence.

Important Elements of Holistic Healing

We shall examine the following essential elements of holistic treatment:

- Physical health: Techniques for preserving and enhancing physical well-being, such as diet, exercise, and pain relief.

- Techniques for managing emotions, lowering stress levels, and promoting emotional equilibrium.

- Mental health: Techniques for improving mental clarity, controlling ideas and beliefs, and maintaining a good outlook.

- Exploring your spiritual habits and beliefs can help you achieve inner calm and a connection to a higher purpose.

- Recognizing how your social connections and environment affect your general well-being and making the necessary adjustments to improve them.

Making Your Comprehensive Healing Plan

We will assist you in developing a specialized holistic health plan that takes into consideration your particular requirements, objectives, and preferences. To encourage balance and well-being, you'll learn how to incorporate several holistic practices into your daily life.

You'll have a thorough grasp of holistic healing by the end of this chapter, along with a plan for putting its ideas into practice in your own life. Join us on this integration journey as we develop a life that respects the interdependence of your body, mind, and emotions, resulting in a more centered and peaceful living.

Creating a Holistic health plan

Developing a customized holistic health plan necessitates careful evaluation of individual needs, goals, and preferences. Here is a generic framework for creating such a strategy that can be tailored to unique requirements:

- Step 1: Establish Clear Goals and Objectives

Begin by establishing specific and attainable health objectives. Weight management, stress reduction, improved fitness, treating a chronic condition, or boosting emotional well-being are some examples. Having specific goals can help guide the creation of your overall strategy.

- Step 2: Evaluate Your Current Health and Lifestyle

Conduct a self-evaluation to better understand your current health and lifestyle. Take into account things like food, exercise, sleep, stress levels, and emotional well-being. It is critical to identify areas that require improvement.

Chapter 14

Resilience and Self-Care

Nurturing Your Mind and Body

We now turn our attention to resilience and self-care, an investigation of how to nourish your mind and body to build resilience against life's obstacles, as we continue our investigation of the deep relationship between emotions, muscles, and general well-being.

The quality of resilience is the capacity to overcome hardship and keep one's sense of well-being. It's a critical component of both your physical and emotional health, and improving your resilience is mostly dependent on self-care.

We will explore the ideas of resilience and self-care in this chapter, as well as how they relate to your muscles and emotions, and we'll look at some useful techniques for developing resilience and making self-care a priority in your life.

Understanding Resilience

The ability to adapt constructively to hardship, stress, or trauma is referred to as resilience. It is about facing life's difficulties with courage and endurance. The link between resilience, muscles, and emotions is complex:

- Physical Resilience: A healthy body, particularly strong muscles, serves as a basis for resilience. Emotional strength is aided by physical well-being.

- Emotional Resilience: Resilient people have greater emotional management, which helps lessen the impact of stress on muscles.

The Importance of Self-Care

Self-care entails taking purposeful steps to prioritize your physical and emotional well-being. It is an essential practice for developing and maintaining resilience.

In this chapter, we'll look at self-care techniques that help boost your mental and physical resilience:

- Exercise, nutrition, sleep, and relaxation techniques that support your physical well-being are examples of physical self-care.
- Mindfulness, emotional release, and therapy are examples of practices that help emotional regulation and healing.
- Building and sustaining good connections, requesting help when required, and interacting with others are all examples of social self-care.
- Mental Self-Care entails cultivating a positive mindset, minimizing stress, and cultivating mental clarity.

Resilience and Self-Care Strategies That Work

We will present you with practical techniques for incorporating resilience and self-care into your daily life. These tactics will assist you in developing mental and physical strength, reducing the impact of stress, and improving your general well-being.

Join us on this path of resilience and self-care, and let's work together to build a life that is full of strength, well-being, and emotional balance.

Chapter 15

The Journey Ahead

Sustaining Mind-Body Harmony

As we near the end of our exploration into the delicate relationship between emotions, muscles, and overall well-being, we reach a turning point—a reflection on the journey thus far and a look ahead at maintaining mind-body harmony.

In this last chapter, we'll go over the key concepts and techniques you've learned throughout the book. We'll also talk about ways to keep your emotions and muscles in harmony as you continue your journey toward optimal well-being.

Key Insights Recap

We've been on a trip together through several facets of the mind-body relationship throughout this book:

- We looked at how emotions are intertwined with muscle tension and physical wellness.

- We learned how relaxation techniques, stress management, and self-care may help us feel better emotionally and physically.

- We looked into activities like yoga, mindfulness, and breathwork, which help us comprehend the mind-body link better.

- We talked about how important nutrition, exercise, and emotional release are for overall wellness.

- We learned the importance of imagination and self-care in overcoming life's problems.

Maintaining Mind-Body Balance

The journey does not end here; it continues as you use the knowledge and practices you've received in your daily life. Here are some important factors to consider to maintain mind-body harmony:

Make the activities and strategies you've learned a regular part of your daily or weekly routine.

- Self-Compassion: Be gentle and compassionate with yourself as you negotiate life's ups and downs. Self-compassion is an essential component of happiness.

- Continue Learning: Keep an open mind to new thoughts and activities that can help you improve your mind-body connection. There is always more to learn.

- Community and Help: Seek out like-minded people for help, whether through friends, support groups, or professional advice.

Your Ongoing Adventure

This book has given you a road map for understanding and nurturing the complex relationship between your emotions and muscles. It's a journey toward better physical and emotional health that you can continue to take long after these pages are finished.

Keep in mind that you can live a harmonious and balanced life. You can live a life of increased vitality, emotional balance, and general well-being by realizing the significant link between your emotions and muscles, practicing self-care, and cultivating resilience.

Take with you the knowledge, habits, and inspiration you've earned on this journey when you close this book. Accept the continual adventure of maintaining mind-body balance, and may it lead you to a life filled with contentment, joy, and self-discovery.

The trip is yours to continue, and the options are endless.

www.ingramcontent.com/pod-product-compliance
Lightning Source LLC
Chambersburg PA
CBHW081608270726
48661CB00021B/4067